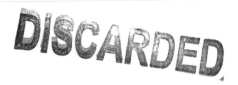

STEROIDS

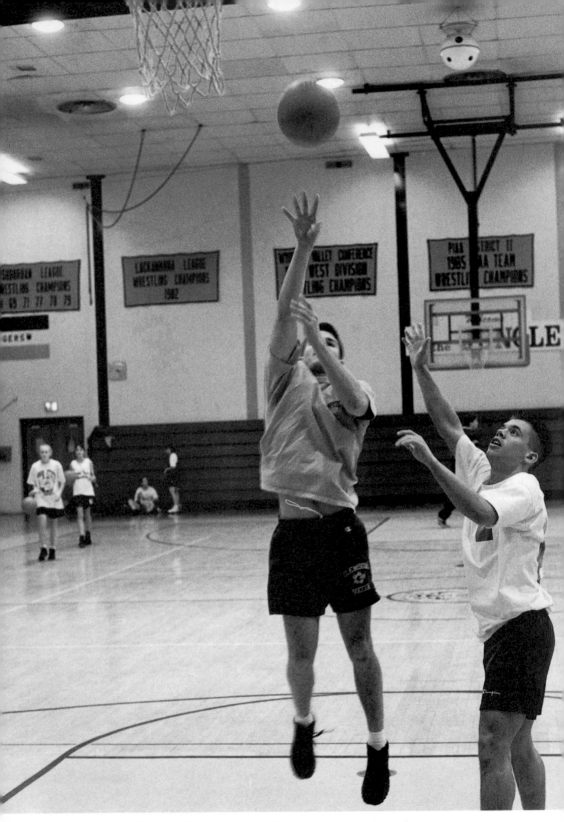

Some athletes use steroids to improve their performance.

THE DRUG ABUSE PREVENTION LIBRARY

STEROIDS

Lawrence Clayton, Ph.D.

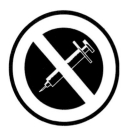

THE ROSEN PUBLISHING GROUP, INC.

NEW YORK

To
Larry, my son,
a great, drug-free athlete.

Published in 1996 by the Rosen Publishing Group, Inc.
29 East 21st Street, New York, NY 10010

First Edition

Library of Congress Cataloging-in-Publication Data

Clayton, L. (Lawrence)
     Steroids / Lawrence Clayton. — 1st ed.
        p.   cm. — (The Drug abuse prevention library)
     Includes bibliographical references (p.   ) and index.
     ISBN 0-8239-2063-1
     1. Doping in sports—Juvenile literature.
     2. Anabolic steroids—Health aspects—Juvenile
literature.   I. Title.   II. Series.
     RC1230.C538   1995
     613.8—dc20   95-1464
                                                                    CIP
                                                                    AC

Manufactured in the United States of America

Contents

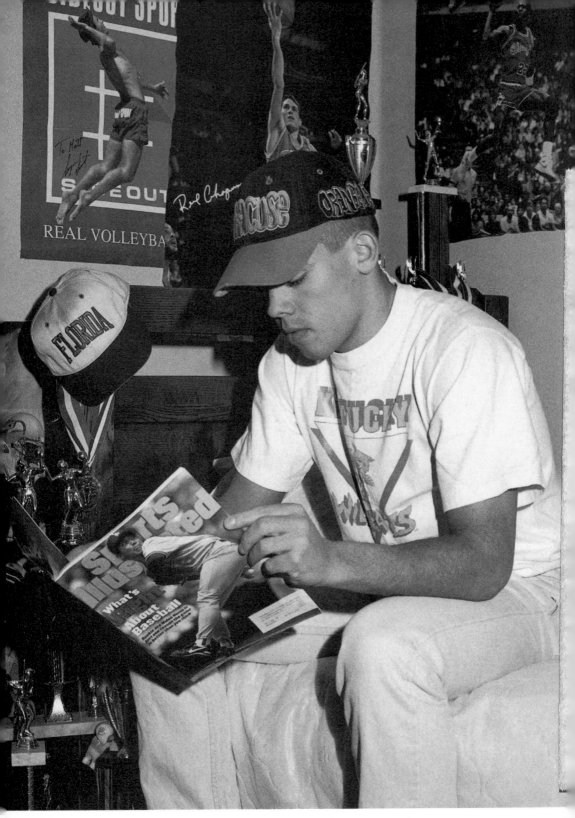

Sports are very important to many people.

CHAPTER 1

The Role of Sports in Your Life

Sports play a very important role in the lives of many young people. You, like most of your friends, probably have favorite teams in several sports: baseball, basketball, and football. You probably have one or more favorite players as well. You may have posters of some of these stars on your bedroom walls. If you're male, you probably collect baseball cards—over half of the boys between the ages of nine and fifteen do—or basketball or football cards.

When you go to the mall, you probably head straight to sporting goods and specialty stores that advertise and sell your favorite pro and college teams' shirts, shoes, shorts, caps, trousers,

8 | bandannas, cups, and pennants.

But sports aren't just for watching. More people your age are playing sports than ever before—some 36 million. They don't just play for their schools, either. They play for the Boys and Girls Clubs of America, the American Legion, the YMCA, Optimist Clubs, and the Little League.

Young people participate in more sports—baseball, softball, swimming, bowling, basketball, football, tennis, track and field, soccer, martial arts, weight lifting, and wrestling—than ever before. They start younger; the average beginning age is just over five. And they are coached by more than 3 million volunteers and 1 million paid coaches.

What do all these statistics mean? What do sports have to offer a person your age?

Sports and Loyalty

One advantage of sports participation is a chance to develop a sense of loyalty. When you play for a team, it becomes more than just a team; it becomes *your* team. You may say, "*We* got creamed" or "*We're* number one!"

Being a part of a team helps you develop a sense of loyalty to things that are bigger than you—your city, state, and country.

Sports and Teamwork

Closely linked to loyalty is the concept of teamwork. Our entire way of life is built on pulling together to achieve something greater than any one person could do.

Consider: We wouldn't have a single car, highway, school, food product, television set, computer, telephone, newspaper, book, airplane, or any of the millions of other things you and I take for granted, without teamwork.

Sports and Fair Play

A sense of fair play is another value that sports provide. When you were a kid— say, six or seven—you didn't understand the idea of fair play. You wanted what you wanted when you wanted it. Fairness had nothing to do with it.

As you got older, the idea of fair play became increasingly important. Now you want an A when you do A-level work. You're upset if someone else gets an A by cheating. You'll feel the same way when you have a job. You'll want to be promoted when you do good work. You'll

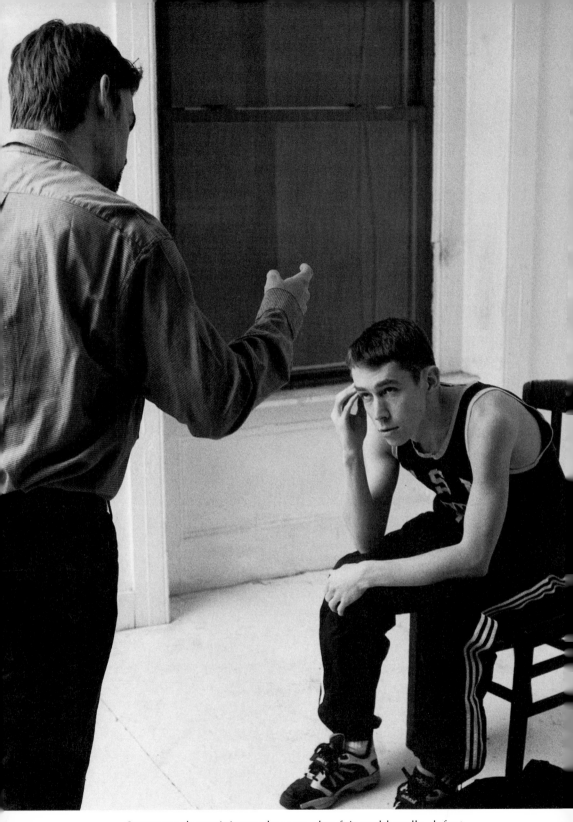

Sports teach participants how to play fair and handle defeat.

be angry if someone else is promoted
because he or she is a manager's relative.

Sports and Sportsmanship

Closely related to fair play is sportsmanship. Sports participation teaches this
value better than any other experience.
You learn to lose the game, but not your
temper or your dignity. You learn to
take a knock-down and get up without
retaliating.

After every game, the opposing
coaches and players shake hands. These
people have just finished doing everything
they could to beat each other. Now they
shake hands. That is sportsmanship. If
you have it, it will color the way you live
your life.

Someday you may want something
badly and not get it. It may be a job or a
dance or a date. When you fail to get it,
what will you do? Remembering what you
learned about sportsmanship will help.

Sports and the Family

Sports offer you a chance to get closer
to your family and to participate in an
activity with them. They support and
console you when your game is off and
cheer you on when you do well. At least,

12 | that's the way it's supposed to be, and in most families, it is.

Other families exert great pressure on teenage sons and daughters to perform, and perform well! You'll see them at any sporting event—parents who seem to hate their teenager because he or she lost the match, struck out, missed a play, or dropped the ball. They are the exception, but they do exist. Some young people want so desperately not to disappoint their families that they will do almost anything, including taking steroids, to succeed.

Sports and Drugs

As important as sports participation is in the lives of young people, it's easy to see why some would do almost anything to become better athletes.

Some have even taken drugs to become bigger, faster, and stronger. They think these drugs are a shortcut to fame and glory. Instead, they are a shortcut to the hospital, the prison, and sometimes the graveyard.

This book is about one class of those drugs, steroids. Teenagers are abusing them in record numbers.

CHAPTER 2

A Short History of Steroid Abuse

*I*n July 1988, a subcommittee of the Judiciary Committee of the U.S. House of Representatives held a hearing on crime. This body hears only issues of the most serious national importance. But there they were, our Representatives and experts from around the country—sports doctors, coaches, athletes, and representatives of the National Football League (NFL), the International Olympic Committee (IOC), the American Medical Association (AMA), the National Collegiate Athletic Association (NCAA), and many more—discussing steroid abuse.

The NFL representative read a statement that said in part, "Anabolic steroids are well worth congressional concern. It

14 | has become clear that they pose numerous and serious medical risks."

Dr. William Howard, chief physician at the Sports Medicine Clinic of Union Memorial Hospital, said that as many as 50 percent of professional athletes were taking steroids to enhance their performance.

Some were even taking steroids that were intended only for race horses. Several were taking twice the amount that would be medically safe for a horse. They were making themselves sick, and some had died.

The Strange Beginnings

How did this happen? How did steroid abuse reach such unhealthy levels?

It started in a most peculiar way. In 1771, John Hunter transplanted the testes of a rooster into a hen. The result was that the hen became more "rooster-like" in appearance and behavior.

The next experiment was more than 100 years later, in 1889, when Dr. Charles E. Brown-Sequard injected himself with testicular extract. He reported feeling stronger and smarter and having improved digestion.

In 1935, scientists discovered that

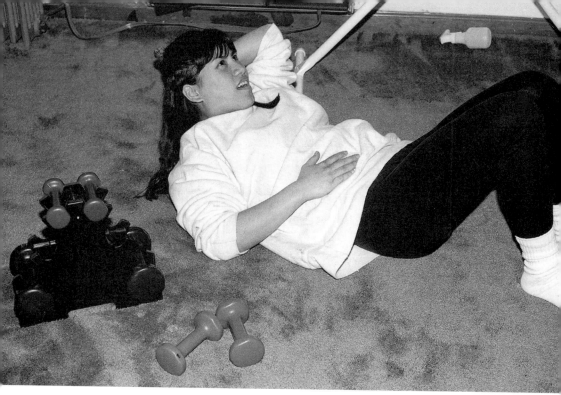

Athletes may try steroids when they feel that physical training isn't enough.

testosterone was the chemical that caused males to be male. From then on, people were interested in finding out just how strong testosterone could make a person.

The idea that drugs could enhance performance was not new. Athletes had been using amphetamines (speed) and other drugs for this purpose for many years, and there had been many casualties.

A Dutch cyclist died in 1986 after being doped with cocaine and heroin by his coach. This caused several sporting organizations to require athletes to be examined for drugs by doctors.

16 | *Athletes Join the Parade*

Weight lifters from the former Soviet Union began using steroids in 1950. Because of this, they dominated all weight-lifting competition for many years. In 1954, the United States Olympic team's physician, Dr. John B. Ziegler, gave steroids to his team, hoping to help them compete with the Soviets.

By 1957, drug use was so widespread that the American Medical Association (AMA) established a group now called the Committee on the Medical Aspects of Sports in a vain attempt to control athletes' drug abuse. Other countries followed suit.

Despite this, a Danish cyclist died at the 1960 Olympic Games from use of amphetamines. In 1967, a French and an English cyclist died from drug abuse. This caused the IOC to begin testing athletes for drugs. In one year, eight cyclists in Winnipeg, two cyclists in Rome, and 17 percent of the Italian soccer team tested positive for drugs.

When drug testing was announced at the world championships in 1970, one athlete dropped out immediately and three others tested positive. At the World Weight-Lifting Championships that year,

nine weight lifters were tested; eight
showed evidence of drug use.

Olympic Drug Tests

In 1972, the IOC began full-scale drug
testing. As a result, four athletes lost
medals they had won, and seven others
were banned from the Games forever.

Anabolic steroids were officially
banned by the IOC in 1975. Even so, the
next year two male weight lifters and one
female discus thrower were disqualified.
Eight others were banned that summer in
Montreal. In 1983, the IOC added caffeine
and testosterone to the list of banned
substances, and the U.S. Food and Drug
Administration banned the production of
Dianabol (a steroid). Diuretics (drugs to
increase the output of urine) and certain
forms of corticosteroids were added to
the list of banned chemicals in 1985.

Brian Bosworth, All-American defensive back of the University of Oklahoma,
was banned from postseason play for
steroid abuse by the NCAA in 1986. The
next year, the NFL checked for steroids
and gave a thirty-day suspension to anyone who tested positive.

In May 1987, the U.S. Department of
Justice filed 100-count indictments

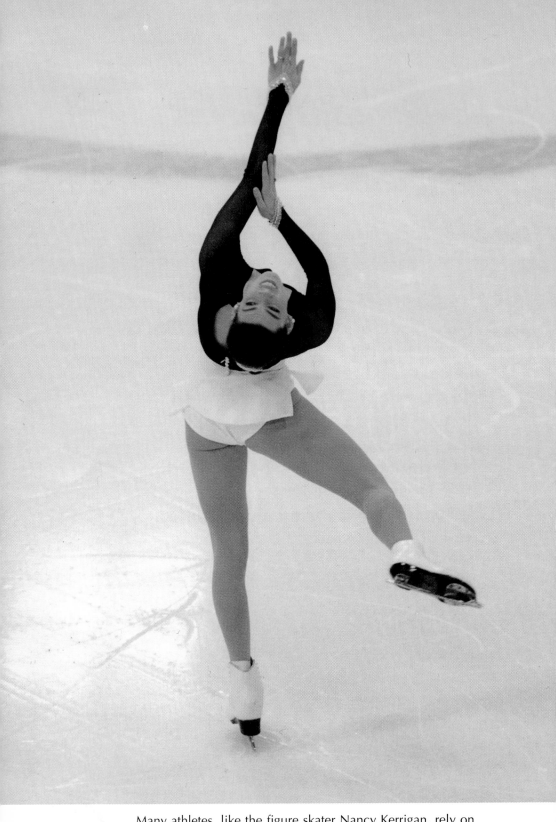

Many athletes, like the figure skater Nancy Kerrigan, rely on their natural strength and talent and stay drug-free.

against thirty-four persons for sale and distribution of anabolic steroids. In the same year, the IOC discovered that some athletes were still using steroids during the off-season, so they began "out-of-competition" drug testing.

At the 1988 Summer Olympics, the world's fastest runner, Canadian Ben Johnson, won a gold medal but was stripped of it and ousted from the Games after he tested positive for steroids.

Steroid Epidemic

By that time, it was clear that a new drug epidemic had struck. It was also clear that it was fueled by anabolic steroids.

That is how the U.S. House of Representatives got involved. At the end of the hearing, steroids were placed under the same restrictions as heroin and cocaine.

Despite this, in 1989 the National Institute on Drug Abuse (NIDA) reported that adolescent steroid use had risen to 4.7 percent of males and 1.3 percent of females. A year later, the U.S. Inspector General reported that adolescent abuse of steroids continued to climb to 11 percent of males and 3 percent of females. That is about 500,000 teenagers. The NCAA

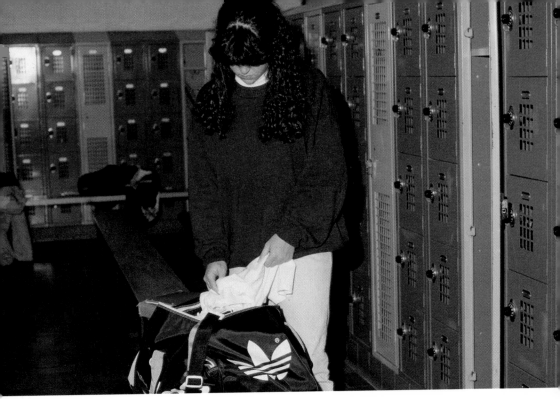

Steroid abuse occurs among both male and female athletes.

joined the IOC in performing intensive drug testing of its athletes.

The Anabolic Steroids Control Act of 1990 set severe penalties for both sale and possession of steroids. The fine for sale was set at $250,000 for the first offense and $500,000 for the second offense. Simple possession can carry a $1,000 fine.

Today, the NIDA estimates that more than 1 million adolescents are steroid users. They support a $100 million trade in black market steroids.

CHAPTER 3

Types of Steroids

*T*he human body contains some 600 different steroids, but there are only three main types. This chapter discusses the medical use and the abuse potential of each type of steroid.

Corticosteroids
Corticosteroids are medically used to control inflammation and pain. They have little potential for abuse.

Estrogenic Steroids
These steroids are made from the female sex hormone estrogen and are used for birth control and as estrogen replacement after the ovaries have been removed or

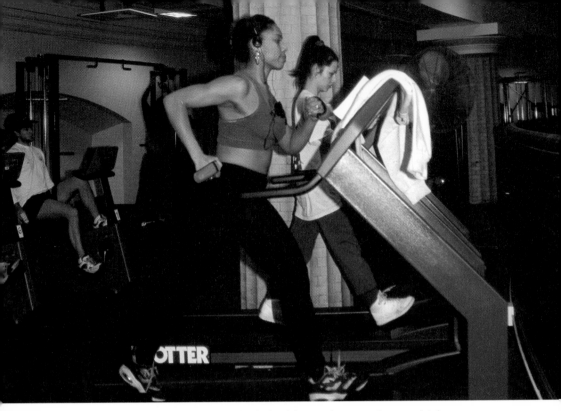

Anabolic steroids, which build muscle tone, have a high potential for abuse.

ceased functioning. They have no potential for abuse.

Anabolic Steroids

Anabolic steroids are made from the male sex hormone (testosterone) and are used medically, *in limited dosages*, for patients with diseases such as cancer or AIDS. They increase muscle and tendon strength for patients who cannot recover naturally. They have an extremely high potential for abuse.

People use anabolic steroids to build
muscle and enhance their performance. It

might take a teenage boy a year of intensive weight lifting to add thirty pounds of muscle to his body. Anabolic steroids, taken in huge amounts, can do it in twelve weeks. Of course, the side effects can be deadly.

The chart below gives the generic and brand names of some of the most common anabolic steroids and how each is administered.

Common Anabolic Steroids

Generic Name	Brand Name	Administration
Calusterone	Methosarb	Oral
Danazol	Danocrine, Danol, Cyclomen, Danatrol, Danobrin, Ladogar, Winobanin	Oral
Dromostandolone	Masteril, Masterone, (Drostanolone) Metormon	Injectable
Proplonate	Permastril, Drolban	Oral
Ethylestrenol	Maxibolin, Orabolin, Otgabolin	
Fluoxymesterone	Android-F, Halotestin, Oralsterone, Oratestin, Ora-Testryl, Ultandren	Oral
Formebolone	Esiclene, Hubernol	Injectable
Furazabol	Miotolone	Oral and Injectable
Mebolazine	Roxilon	Oral
Mesterolone	Mestoranum, Proviron	Oral
Methandriol	Sinsex, Stenediol, Troformone	Oral

24

Generic Name	Brand Name	Administration
Methandrostenolone (Methandienone)	Andoredan, Danabol, Dianabol, Encephan, Lanabolin, Metabolina, Metaboline, Metanabol, Metastenol, Nerobol, Perbolin	Oral and Injectable
Methenolone	Primobolan, Primobolan Despot, Primobolan S, Primonbol	Oral and Injectable
Methyltestosterone	Androyd, Glosso-Sterandryl, Mesteron, Metandren, Neo-Hombreol, Neohombreol-M, Methyltestosterone Orchisterone, Oreton, Methyl, Primotest, Testin, Testomet, Testovis, Testred, Virilon, Virormone-Oral	Oral
Mibolerone	Nilevar	Oral
Nandrolone	Anobolin LA-100, Androlone Hybolin Deconoate, Kabolin, Nandrolin, Neo-Durabolic	Injectable
Oxabolone	Steranabol Despot, Steranabol Ritardo	Injectable
Oxandrolone	Anavar, Antitriol, Lonavar	Oral
Oxymesterone	Anamidol, Balinmax, Oranabol, Oranabol-10	Oral
Oxymetholone	Anapolon-50, Androl 50, Adroyd,	Oral

Generic Name	Brand Name	Administration	*25*
	Anadroyd, Anasterone, Anasteronal, Nastenon, Oxitosona-50, Pardroyd, Plenastril, Synasteron, Zenalosyn		
Quinbolone	Anabolicum Vister	Oral	
Stanozolol	Winstrol, Anasyth, Stromba, Strombajeck, Winstrol	Oral	
Testosterone	Androil, Anadronate, BayTestone, Depo-Testrosterone, Jectatest-LA, Malogen LA, Sustanon, Restandol, Testate, Testone LA, Testostroval	Oral and Injectable	
Trenbolone	Parabolan, Finajet, Finaplix	Injectable	

These drugs are available only by prescription. Some, such as Dianabol, are used only for horses and are not even available by prescription.

Drug dealers do a huge black market business selling anabolic steroids. The U.S. Food and Drug Administration estimates that $600,000 dollars' worth of all illegal steroid sales take place through private fitness centers and

26 | gymnasiums every year. That's about 79
percent of all the steroids sold in the
United States.

CHAPTER 4

What Steroids Do to Your Body

*S*teroids change your body in many ways. Some of the changes affect everyone; others affect only males. Still others affect only females. Most of the changes are negative, but there are a few positives.

Positive Changes
Steroids do help healing and increase strength. Doctors prescribe them for patients who have been seriously injured or are gravely ill. However, doctors usually give them as a last resort, and even then, only in very small doses.

Steroids have dangerous side effects. Whereas the positive effects of steroid

28 abuse fade away when use is stopped, the side effects tend to be permanent.

Side Effects That Can Strike Boys

Steroid abuse makes males look more like females. It causes unusual breast development and shrinking and drying up of the testicles.

Other side effects are impotence, swelling of the prostate gland to the point of needing to be catheterized (process in which a hollow tube is used to drain fluids) to urinate, and severe penis pain.

Side Effects That Can Strike Girls

Steroid abuse makes females look more like males, causing them to grow facial and body hair and develop male-pattern baldness, deepening of the voice, menstrual problems, and clitoral enlargement.

The fetal damage that can result in birth defects may be the most devastating effect of steroid use by pregnant women.

Side Effects That Can Strike Anyone

Although you will not get every one of these problems if you choose to use steroids, you will experience many of the side effects.

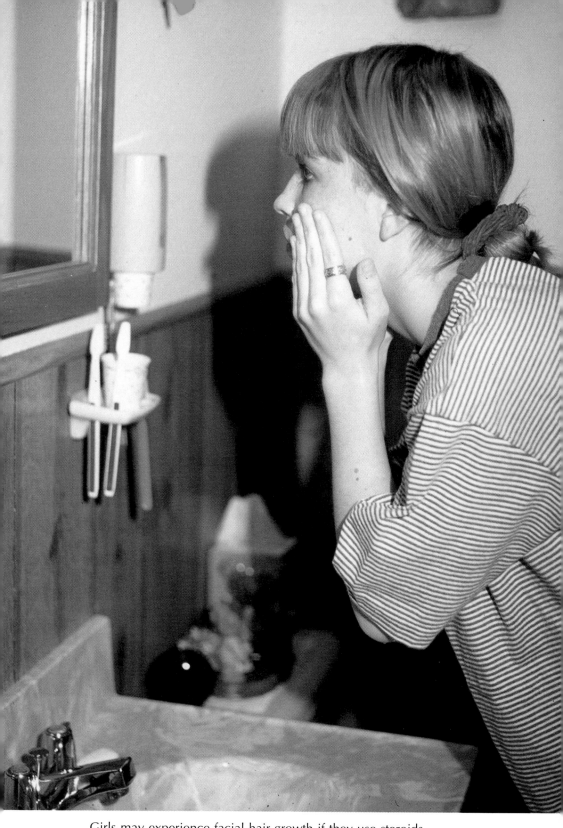

Girls may experience facial hair growth if they use steroids.

30 | *Skin Problems*

Steroid abuse wreaks havoc with the skin, the body's largest organ. It causes:

Extremely oily skin. People who use steroids often look as if they've been working at an auto lubrication station, because their clothes get so oily. Any dirt in the air sticks to them, and by the end of the day ring-around-the-collar is very evident.

Hives. Many people have an allergic reaction to steroids that causes hives, a horribly itchy rash. Some people also get purple spots on the head, neck, and body.

Severe acne. Teenagers are subject to acne, but steroid abusers get a very severe kind that is deep below the surface of the skin. It often becomes inflamed and erupts into huge pus- and blood-filled pimples that take a long time to heal. When they do heal, they frequently leave permanent scars on a person's face, neck, chest, and back.

Coronary Artery Problems

Steroids cause changes in the body that set the abuser up for coronary artery problems. A blood analysis often looks as if it came from someone very old. It shows high levels of everything bad—high blood pressure, high cholesterol, high numbers of sugar and fat cells. Steroids also weaken the heart, which leads to such problems as heart attack, stroke, and premature senility. Most steroid abusers die long before they should.

Take Steve Courson, former linebacker for the Pittsburgh Steelers and the Tampa Bay Buccaneers, as an example. His doctor has told him that he is dying from heart failure because of steroid abuse. Ask Steve if the few years of glory were worth it. He'll tell you in a minute, "Don't mess with steroids. They're killers."

Liver and Kidney Problems

Steroids are particularly hard on the liver, making it unable to clear the blood of poisons. This causes jaundice, a yellowing of the eyes and skin. It also frequently causes liver tumors.

Steroids attack the kidneys, causing them to malfunction and eventually to fail. As the kidneys grow weaker, they are unable to do their job of eliminating excess water from the body. This water retention gives steroid abusers a bloated look and causes their legs and feet to swell.

32 | *Muscle and Bone Problems*

The liver, kidney, and heart problems caused by steroids eventually cause the muscles to cramp painfully. Muscle and tendon injuries become frequent. Bones begin to ache in various parts of the body.

A problem that is especially damaging to teenagers is premature maturation; that is, the body becomes mature before it should. A twelve-year-old may develop large muscles and a beard and start going bald. Growth plates in his bones close forever so that he can never grow taller. By the time he's fourteen, all the other boys are bigger and stronger. By the time he's sixteen, he is too small to compete at all.

Internal Problems

Steroids mess up the internal organ systems. Abusers often feel nauseated and sometimes vomit blood. They have diarrhea, chills, tongue pain, and permanent bad breath.

They may experience fainting, dizziness, and fatigue. Steroids can also cause blood poisoning, gallstones, and cancer.

Other Complications

Steroid abuse can cause epileptic-like seizures (uncontrolled, involuntary con-

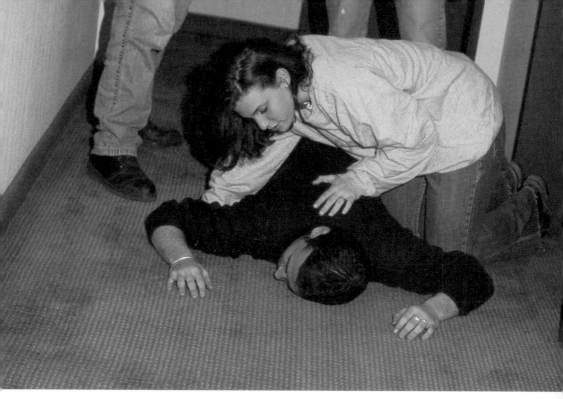

Steroid abusers may suffer from seizures.

vulsions), which sometimes result in
death. Most abusers suffer insomnia
(inability to sleep) and severe headaches.

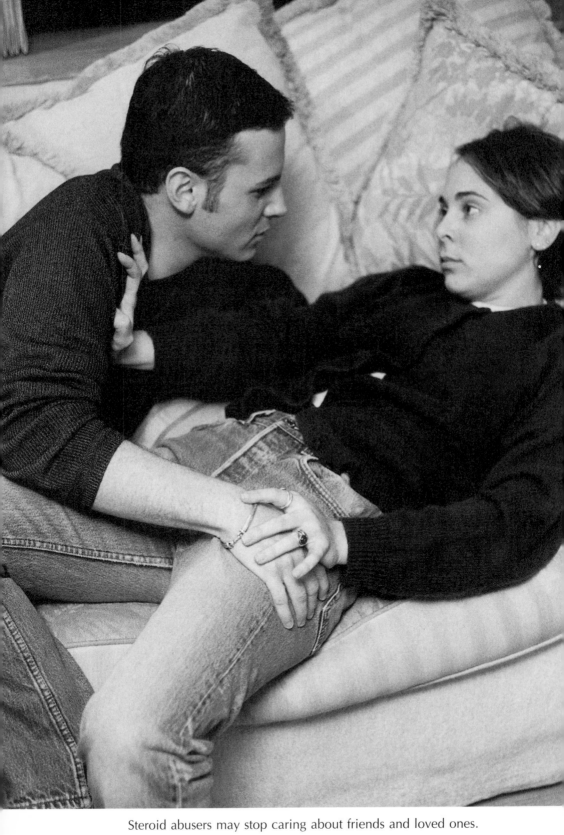

Steroid abusers may stop caring about friends and loved ones.

CHAPTER 5

How Steroids Change Your Personality

*S*teroids change your personality in very specific ways, all undesirable. Some are so dangerous that they could cost you your life or cause you to take someone else's!

They can make you self-centered, egotistical, and inconsiderate. They can make you angry, aggressive, and violent— perhaps homicidal. Sometimes they make you depressed and even suicidal.

Steroids Can Make You Self-Centered

Steroid abuse really messes up your mind. Users become "stuck on themselves." Little by little, family, friends, teammates—even girlfriends or boyfriends—mean less and less to them. Eventually they get to the point where

35

36 | only their own desires are important. Other people become just things to use to make the abuser happy.

Ricky

Everyone said that Ricky was an athlete with promise. In both elementary and middle school, he had lettered in four sports. Now, as a freshman, he seemed destined to do the same in high school.

He had been dating Lori for two years. One evening, after a football game, he and Lori were sitting in her mom's car. Lori kissed him, and he kissed her back. Nothing unusual there. But his kisses became hard and demanding. Lori, frightened, said, "We'd better stop!"

Instead, Ricky put his hand inside her blouse and under her bra. "Don't!" shouted Lori in a panic.

"Shut up," said Ricky.

"But you promised you wouldn't push me," cried Lori.

"So who cares?" he snarled as he pushed her down and forced himself on top of her.

Just then, her father opened the car door and pulled Ricky off Lori.

In Lori's living room she explained to their parents what had happened. Turning to Ricky, she said, "I've never been so afraid in my life!"

Ricky just glared at her and said, "Tell it | **37**
to somebody who cares."

"Ricky!" shouted his mother. "What's
happened to you?"

"Screw you," Ricky said coldly.

With that, his father walked over to Ricky
and said, "Son, your mother and I think you
have been abusing steroids. Maybe you're
even addicted to them."

Sounding bored, Ricky said, "Get a life,
Dad."

"You're the one who needs to get a life,
son," said his father. "You're either going to
treatment or to jail. Which will it be?"

"Jail!" Ricky sneered.

"You got it," said his father.

Three weeks later, Ricky was standing
in front of the juvenile court judge for
sentencing.

"You are guilty of the attempted rape of
Lori Paxton. Your sentence is four years in
the Juvenile Detention Center. If, during
your stay, you successfully complete treatment
for steroid addiction, this court will consider
reducing your sentence."

Steroid abuse seriously damages your
ability to care about others. Many steroid
abusers report feeling very alone. They
become self-centered and insensitive.

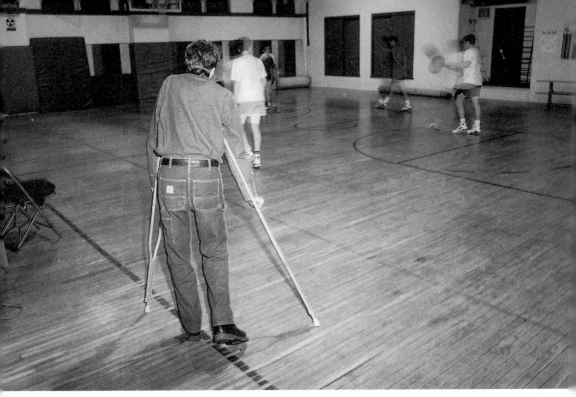

As well as causing physical problems, steroids can make athletes angry and violent.

Steroids Can Make You Angry

Another way steroids mess with your mind is that they cause you to be unreasonably angry—sometimes at those you most love, sometimes at total strangers. For some, the consequences are serious, perhaps life-threatening.

Bonju

Bonju was big. He was the best defensive back anyone at Valley North had ever seen. He was looking forward to a great college career and maybe even becoming a pro after that. Then Valley North's coach got a better job offer and Valley North got a new coach.

At his first meeting with the players, **39**
Coach Dennis instituted a new policy:
random drug testing. "No player of mine is
going to mess up his life with drugs," he said.
"And no team of mine is going to win a
championship because of something artificial.
We win ours the old-fashioned way—by being
better than our competition! So, anybody on
steroids, stop now. If you don't and you get
caught, you're off the team. It's that simple."

Bonju just laughed. The coach wouldn't
throw him off the team.

Then one day Coach Dennis walked up to
Bonju after practice and handed him a small
paper cup. Motioning toward the team
trainer, he said, "Give the man a sample."

A week later, the coach called Bonju into
his office. "Bonju, your test came back; you're
positive and you're out of here," he said.

Bonju couldn't believe it. "Throwing me
off the team? That's ridiculous. I'll talk to the
principal."

Angrily, he stormed out of the school and
to the parking lot. Jumping into his Camaro,
he took off with tires squealing. The police
estimated that he was going well over 100
miles per hour when he hit the Toyota, killing
a family of four.

The papers said that Bonju was luckier
than the family he killed—but you might

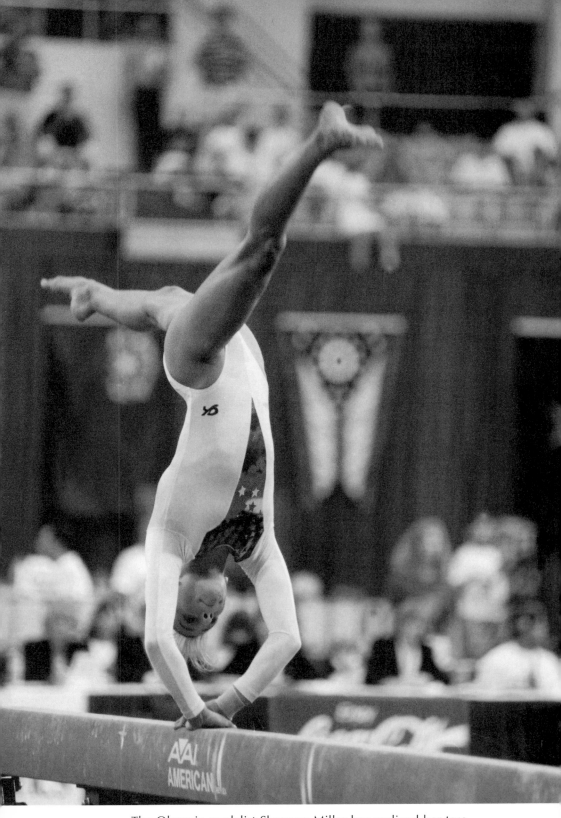

The Olympic medalist Shannon Miller has realized her true potential without help from drugs.

want to ask him. His back was broken in the wreck. He'll spend the rest of his life in a wheelchair.

Of course, not all steroid abusers experience such a tragedy, but do you want to take that chance? Do you want some chemical deciding your reactions? Shouldn't that be your choice?

Steroids Make You Violent

People who abuse steroids can become violent in a flash. This makes them unpredictable and untrustworthy, and having them as friends can be dangerous and perhaps deadly.

Sherry

Sherry had never felt like part of the crowd. She felt alone, left out. She wanted desperately to be popular.

She would have liked to play sports, but she was too short and small to be any good at basketball or volleyball, her school's biggest girls' sports. "It's no use," she told herself. "I'll never be good at anything."

Then one day Shannon Miller, the Olympic medalist, spoke to the student body during assembly. Right away Sherry liked her. Shannon was short, just like her. When

42 | she talked about her life, she said that she had always felt left out but that gymnastics had changed all that. After her speech, the students gave Shannon a standing ovation. Now Sherry knew exactly what she would do. Gymnastics could change her life just as it had changed Shannon's.

That very day Sherry enrolled in a gymnastics class, but she found she was too weak to do well, especially her ankles. Then a "friend" from class introduced her to steroids. She started getting stronger right from the beginning.

A year later, she was a much better gymnast. There was even talk of putting her on the team. Sherry was delighted. "You need more work on the balance beam, Sherry," said Cindy, another gymnast. "You'll never make the team like that."

"I'm better than you!" shouted Sherry.

"I was only trying to help," said Cindy. "I thought you . . ."

Sherry began screaming and cursing. "You jerk, who appointed you God?" Then Sherry hit her. Not once, but over and over. She was like a wild person. It took the coach and several other athletes to subdue her. Cindy had to be hospitalized.

Needless to say, Sherry was suspended from school. But the worst came three days *later when she showed up for practice. The coach said, "Sherry, we don't need you here. You're bad news, kid. Trouble. You need help. Find yourself a therapist!"*

43

"Roid rage" has been known to cause steroid abusers to commit murder. The girl Sherry attacked was lucky to be alive. And Sherry was lucky that she didn't go to jail.

Steroids Can Make You Depressed

Abuse of steroids is so hard on the body that the abuser eventually has to stop using them or die. Those who do stop become seriously depressed. Mental health professionals call this kind of depression steroid-induced anhedonia. It means a period of time when everything loses its meaning and joy: sports, friends, family, being big and strong, even life itself. It could also be called steroid withdrawal. By whatever name, it is horrible to experience.

Jerry

Jerry Johnson's father said he was "too sensitive for his own good," but Jerry was one of those "gentle souls" who really care about others. He wouldn't steal a base because

44   *"sliding in might hurt someone." He didn't like hunting or fishing because "killing an animal or a fish when you aren't even hungry is cruel."*

One day when Mr. Johnson was driving to work he heard a newscaster on the radio say that one of the side effects of steroid abuse was aggressiveness. "Just what Jerry needs," he thought. That evening he stopped at the gym and asked a trainer about steroids.

"No problem," said the trainer. "You look like you're in pretty good physical health. I could inject you, myself . . ."

"I'll let my wife do that," he said. "She's a nurse."

And that was it. Soon he was giving the injections to Jerry, and the boy did become more aggressive. In fact, in less than six months he had put on thirty pounds and was on the varsity football team.

Then one day, his wife called him at work sounding frantic.

"Jerry is having chest pain and his blood pressure is sky-high," she said, panicked. "I'm taking him to the hospital. Meet us there."

By the time he arrived, he found Jerry in the emergency room, with doctors and nurses working feverishly over him.

His wife said, "The doctor says that

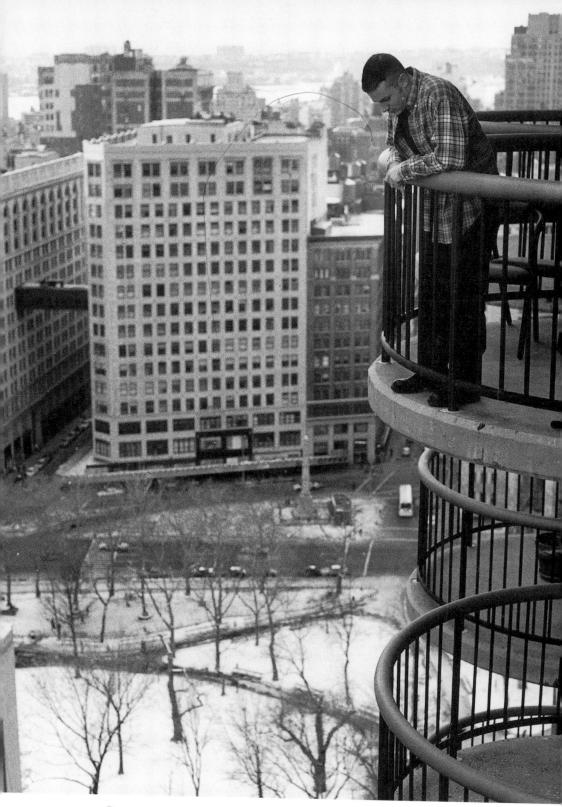

Depression caused by steroid withdrawal can lead some former users to commit suicide.

46 | *he's on steroids, almost ten times the usual dosage! Where on earth would he get something like that?"*

Jerry's life was saved that evening. He was able to come home a week later, and the whole family thought their life would return to normal.

Six weeks later, Jerry was once again admitted to the hospital, this time with deep depression. He had been found sitting in his car in the school parking lot, unable to muster the energy even to get out.

That's what can happen to steroid abusers when they quit. They become so depressed that they may need medical assistance to deal with the simplest things. Even then, it can take a long time to get over it completely.

Steroids Can Make You Suicidal

Some steroid abusers don't get over their use. The depression is so severe that they just can't cope, and they end up taking their own lives.

Ellen

Ellen never seemed to have any choices in her life. People were always deciding everything for her. It started when she was six years old. Her father was working as a clerk in a grocery store when a man pointed a gun at him and ordered him to open the cash register. Just then, a police car pulled up. The robber panicked and pulled the trigger, killing her father instantly.

Five months later, her mother married another man. Ellen hated him right from the beginning, but she didn't have a vote. Her mother simply showed up one day with a fat man who was smelly and always sweating. "This is Tom," she announced. "He's your new stepdad."

Then her mother got sick. Cancer, they said. After the surgery came months of chemotherapy. When her mother wasn't in the hospital, she was sick.

It was during this time that Tom started sexually abusing Ellen. No vote here either. He put it to her this way: "If you don't go along, I'll divorce your mother. She can't work. She'll lose the house and the car, and you'll both be on the street. It's up to you."

Ellen got pregnant when she was thirteen. "You can't raise a baby at your age," said her mother. And that settled it. When the baby was born, she had to put it up for adoption. No one asked what Ellen wanted. She wasn't given a choice.

In her junior year, Ellen started dating

48 *Gene, the discus thrower on the school track team. She watched him practice almost every evening. One day he said, "Give it a try." Without even thinking, Ellen whirled the discus as she'd seen Gene do and let go. It sailed so far, it looked like a frisbee. "Hey!" shouted her boyfriend, "that was an incredible toss!" Turning toward the fieldhouse, he yelled, "Hey, Coach! You gotta see this!"*

The coach trotted toward them. "How far did she throw it?"

"Looks like 118 feet, nine inches," Gene said.

"Holy cow!" said the coach. "Are you kidding? That's just eight feet off the school record!"

Soon Ellen was on the girls' track team. Winning meet after meet, she set a new school record. Then she came up against Julie Rosco from Peabody. Julie's first toss was 130 feet, two inches. Ellen knew she wasn't that strong. Still, she gave it her best shot— 126 feet, six inches—good enough for second place. Her coach said, "Second's OK, but you'll have to get a lot stronger to take State!"

When Gene suggested steroids, Ellen went along with it. Soon she was being injected with Parabolan, a powerful steroid. She got stronger fast. Her discus tosses were better and better. By the time State came, she won it easily, beating Julie by six feet and setting a new state record of 142 feet, three inches.

A month later, Gene told her that he wanted to date other girls.

"But I won State," Ellen cried. "Isn't that what you wanted?"

He just looked away and said, "You may have won State, but you look like a freak!"

That night, Ellen stood in front of the mirror in her bathroom. She was looking at her huge muscles and her dark mustache as she raised the gun to her head. "He's right," she said. "At least, this will be my choice." And she pulled the trigger.

Her mother blamed her illness. Her friends blamed her boyfriend. Her stepfather blamed himself. Her boyfriend blamed Ellen. The Medical Examiner blamed the steroids.

Even though the worst of the depression is usually over in three to six months, steroid-induced anhedonia can last as long as five years.

CHAPTER 6

People Who Can Help

*F*ew things can mess up your life more or faster than steroid abuse. If you or someone you care about is hooked on steroids, you will probably need help to stop or get them to stop.

Steroids are too dangerous to stop using without medical help. Many people die each year trying to quit using these chemicals. If you have been using steroids for long, here are some people you can turn to for help.

Your Parents

You may be surprised that the list begins with your parents. Some teenagers are.

Parents almost always want to help, and they are usually good helpers when

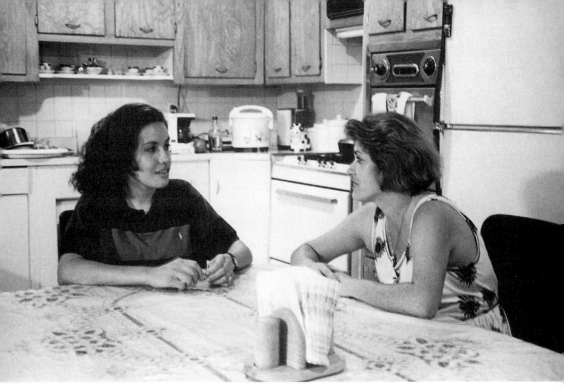

Give your parents a chance to help you kick a steroid habit.

given the chance. Most parents really care about their kids. Sure, they may be shocked to discover that you are abusing steroids, but they've been shocked before. They will get over it. When they do, most of them can be counted on to do their best for you. You might start by giving them this book to read.

If your parents can't or won't help, don't give up. The important thing is that you get the help you need.

Your Teacher
Most teachers like to help young people. That's part of the reason they became

52 teachers. You probably won't be the first person your teacher has helped with a problem like this.

If your teacher doesn't know exactly what to do, he or she will usually know where to find out. So, ask! If that doesn't work, go to the next person on your list.

Your School Counselor

Counselors are specially trained to help people with problems. It's their job. Many of them know a lot about steroids. Some of them will be acquainted with the services available in the community.

But again, if your school counselor doesn't help, try someone else. Getting help is worth the search.

Minister, Priest, or Rabbi

These professionals can be a great source of help. Many understand addiction and are eager to help. Some may know exactly where to refer you for help. They may also be helpful with the problem of telling your parents. They may even be willing to be with you when you tell them.

A word of warning, however. If your religious leader tells you that prayer alone will get rid of your addiction, find another helper. Remember, you will probably need medical help in getting off steroids.

Crisis and Drug Hot Lines

Larger cities have several telephone counseling services established to help young people. They are staffed by people who understand alcohol and other drugs. They know where the best services are and may even be able to make an appointment and arrange transportation for you to see a doctor.

Some of these services are staffed by peer counselors. These are people your age who have been trained to help others. It may be easier for you to discuss your problem with one of them. In any case, be sure to tell the person who answers the phone everything you can about the types and amounts of steroids you have been using.

The School Nurse

School nurses are trained to recognize and deal with medical issues like addiction. One of the benefits of talking to a nurse is that he or she can help if you need emergency medical care. If you have been trying to get off steroids without medical help (especially if you are already

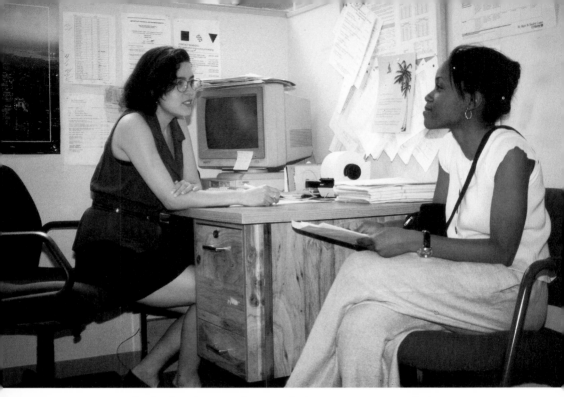

Professional counselors can help users overcome their addiction.

feeling sick or depressed), a school nurse would be an excellent choice.

Certified Alcohol and Drug Counselor (CADC)

CADCs are the professionals in the drug and alcohol field. They spend much of their lives helping people who are addicted. They can help you in more ways than can anyone else.

CADCs are trained to counsel persons who are addicted. They can help you talk to your parents about the problem. They can also help you decide what steps to take to overcome your addiction.

If you are going into withdrawal, they
will recognize the symptoms and get you
the help you need. Because they have
treated many other young people who are
addicted, they can tell you what to expect
as you take the steps to stop using
steroids.

To find a CADC, look in the Yellow
Pages under Alcoholism or Drug
Counselors. You will find the letters CADC
after the counselors' names.

Your Doctor

Another good place to start looking for
help is your family doctor. Doctors are
trained to handle medical problems.
Some are especially good at handling
persons who are in withdrawal from
drugs, including steroids.

Call a doctor at once if you or someone you care about is experiencing any of
the following symptoms: nausea or vomit-
ing, spitting up blood, chest pain, blood
pressure of 140/90 or over, excessive
anger, convulsions, dizziness or fainting,
depression, or suicidal thoughts.

Glossary
Explaining New Words

addict Person who is "hooked" on a drug, or is unable to stop using it.

amphetamines Drugs that excite the mind and body.

anabolic steroids Steroids that build muscle mass.

androgenic steroids Steroids that masculinize: They deepen the voice and cause growth of facial and body hair and male-pattern baldness.

atrophy To dry or shrivel up.

black market Illegal trade.

clitoris Small, sensitive gland at the upper end of the vulva.

corticosteroids Steroids that control inflammation and pain.

diuretic Medication that causes the body to rid itself of excess fluid.

doping   Giving drugs to athletes or race
horses.

drug abuse   Use of a drug in a manner
other than prescribed, or an illegal
drug.

estrogen replacement   Use of a
synthetic female sex hormone as a
replacement for that which the body
has quit producing.

homicidal   Having a tendency toward
murder.

jaundice   Liver disorder that gives a
yellowish cast to the skin and eyes.

male-pattern baldness   Type of baldness typical in older males.

paranoia   Unwarranted suspicion or
fear.

prostate gland   Gland that surrounds
the urethra near its connection to the
bladder in the male.

"roid rage"   Slang term for the unpredictable, psychotic-like behavior
characteristic of steroid abusers.

"stacking"   Slang term for the abuse of
several types of steroids during the
same cycle.

testes   Male reproductive glands.

testosterone   Male sex hormone.

Help List

American College of Sports Medicine
P.O. Box 1440
Indianapolis, IN 46206-1440
(317) 637-9200
web site: http://www.acsm.org/sportsmed

American Council for Drug Education
204 Monroe Street
Rockville, MD 20852
(301) 294-0600

Department of Health and Human Services
Public Health Services, Food and Drug Administration, Office of Public Affairs
5600 Fishers Lane
Rockville, MD 20857
(301) 443-4513
e-mail: NIMHINFO@NIH.GOV

International Certification Reciprocity Consortium
3725 National Drive Suite 213
Raleigh, NC 27612

(919) 781-9734

Narcotic and Drug Research, Inc.
11 Beach Street
New York, NY 10013
(212) 966-8700

National Clearinghouse for Alcohol and Drug Information
P.O. Box 2345
Rockville, MD 20852
(301) 468-2600
web site: http://www.health.org
e-mail: info@prevlane.health.org

National Council on Alcohol and Drug Dependency (NCADD)
12 West 21st Street
New York, NY 10010
(212) 206-6770
(800) 622-2255
web site: http://www.ncadd.org
e-mail: national@NCADD.org

National Drug Abuse Center
5530 Wisconsin Avenue, NW
Washington, DC 20015
(800) 333-2294

60 | Resource Center on Substance Abuse Prevention and Disabilities

1819 L Street, NW, Suite 300
Washington DC 20036
(202) 628-8080
(800) 628-8442

U.S. Department of Justice

Drug Enforcement Administration,
Demand Reduction Section
700 Army/Navy Drive
Arlington, VA 22202
(202) 307-7936

IN CANADA

Alcohol and Drug Dependency Information and Counseling Services (ADDICS)

#2, 2471 1/2 Portage Avenue
Winnipeg, MB R3J 0N6
(204) 831-1999

Youth Detox Program

Family Services Greater Vancouver
504 Cassiar Street
Vancouver, BC V5K 4M9
(604) 299-1131

For Further Reading

Books

Ball, Jacqueline. *Everything You Need to Know About Drug Abuse*, rev. ed. New York: Rosen Publishing Group, 1994.

Berger, George. *The Pressure to Take Drugs*. New York: Watts, 1990.

Bowen-Woodward, Kathy. *Coping with a Negative Body Image*. New York: Rosen Publishing Group, 1989.

Clayton, Lawrence. *Everything You Need to Know About Sports Injuries*. New York: Rosen Publishing Group, 1995.

Edelson, Edward. *Sports Medicine*. New York: Chelsea House, 1988.

Garrick, James, and Radetsky, Peter. *Peak Condition*. New York: Crown, 1986.

Gravits, H., and Bowden, J. *Guide to Recovery*. Holmes Beach, FL: Learning Publications, 1985.

Peck, Rodney. *Drugs and Sports*. New York: Rosen Publishing Group, 1992.

Tuttle, Dave. *Forever Natural—How to Excel in Sports Drug-Free*. Venice, CA: Iron Books, 1990.

Wegscheider, Sharon. *The Miracle of Recovery*. Deerfield Beach, FL: Health Communications, 1989.

62 | Wright, James. *Anabolic Steroids: Altered States*. Carmel, IN: Benchmark, 1990.

Videos

"Anabolic Steroids: The Quest for Superman." Minneapolis: Hourglass Productions, 1990.

"What Price Glory? Myths and Realities of Anabolic Steroids." Edison, NJ: David Thomas Productions, 1989.

Index

64

About the Author

Lawrence Clayton is an International Certified Alcohol and Drug Counselor and president of the Oklahoma Drug and Alcohol Professional Counselor Certification Board. In 1994 he was selected Oklahoma "Counselor of the Year" by the Oklahoma Drug and Alcohol Counselor Association. He lives in Piedmont, Oklahoma, with his wife, Cathy, and their three teenage children.

Photo Credits

p. 15 by Kim Sonsky, pp. 18, 40 © A/P Wide World Photos, p. 22 by Guillermina de Ferrari, pp. 51, 54 by Maria Moreno, all other photos and cover by John Novajosky